MEDITARANEAN DASH DIET COOKBOOK FOR SENIORS

Healthy and delicious recipes to lower high blood pressure and lose excess weight at old age

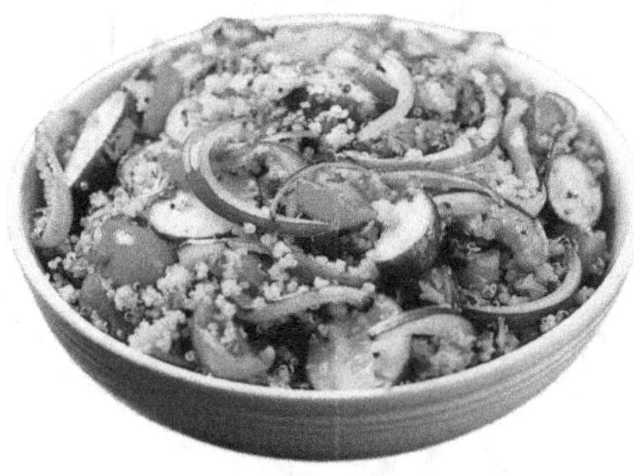

Dr. Malvin Harison

TABLE OF CONTENT

Introduction

Welcome to the flavorful world of the "Mediterranean Dash Diet Cookbook for Seniors" — a culinary journey crafted to nourish both body and soul. This book is a delightful invitation to explore the harmonious fusion of two powerhouse diets renowned for their health benefits – the Mediterranean and DASH (Dietary Approaches to Stop Hypertension) diets.

Designed with seniors in mind, these recipes seamlessly blend the richness of Mediterranean flavors with the heart-healthy principles of the DASH diet. Embark on a gastronomic adventure that not only supports overall well-being but also celebrates the joy of savoring delicious, nutrient-packed meals.

Let this cookbook be your guide to a vibrant, flavorful, and healthful journey through the heart of the Mediterranean and the essence of the DASH diet, tailored to the needs of our beloved seniors.

Understanding the Mediterranean Dash Diet

The Mediterranean Dash Diet Cookbook is your comprehensive guide to unlocking the secrets of two acclaimed diets – the Mediterranean diet and the DASH (Dietary Approaches to Stop Hypertension) diet – tailor-made for seniors. This cookbook is not just a collection of recipes; it's an exploration of the synergies between these two nutritional powerhouses, offering a holistic approach to well-being.

Inside, you'll discover:

1. Flavors of the Mediterranean: Immerse yourself in the richness of Mediterranean cuisine, celebrated for its heart-healthy ingredients, vibrant colors, and tantalizing tastes. From olive oil to fresh herbs, experience the essence of a diet renowned for promoting longevity and vitality.

2. DASHing Towards Health: Uncover the principles of the DASH diet, specifically designed to manage hypertension. Learn how to incorporate nutrient-rich foods, reduce sodium intake, and cultivate habits that support cardiovascular health.

3. Published for Seniors: Recognizing the unique needs of seniors, this cookbook provides recipes that are not only delicious but also address dietary considerations for this stage of life.

Discover meals that are easy to prepare, gentle on the palate, and packed with essential nutrients.

4. A Culinary Journey: Embark on a culinary journey that transcends the realm of mere recipes. Understand the science behind the Mediterranean and DASH diets, and how their combination can offer a holistic approach to health, providing seniors with a roadmap to enhanced well-being.

5. Practical Guidance: Receive practical tips on meal planning, grocery shopping, and maintaining a healthy lifestyle. This cookbook is not just about what's on the plate but also about fostering habits that contribute to long-term health.

Importance of Eating the Right Diet

The importance of taking the right diet is paramount, particularly when considering its impact on overall health and well-being. Here's a general overview of the importance:

1. Nutrient Supply: A well-balanced diet ensures the intake of essential nutrients such as vitamins, minerals, proteins, and healthy fats. These nutrients play vital roles in maintaining bodily functions, supporting the immune system, and promoting optimal organ function.

2. Disease Management: Certain health conditions, like colitis, chronic kidney disease, and Alzheimer's, can benefit from specific dietary approaches. The right diet may help manage symptoms, slow down disease progression, and improve overall quality of life.

3. Energy and Vitality: The right combination of carbohydrates, proteins, and fats provides the energy needed for daily activities. It supports physical endurance, mental alertness, and a general sense of vitality.

4. Digestive Health: A diet rich in fiber from fruits, vegetables, and whole grains supports digestive health. It aids in maintaining regular bowel movements, preventing constipation, and fostering a healthy gut microbiome.

5. Heart Health: Heart-friendly diets, such as the Mediterranean and DASH diets, contribute to cardiovascular health by promoting healthy cholesterol levels, managing blood pressure, and reducing the risk of heart-related diseases.

Complications if the Right Diet is Not Taken

1. Nutrient Deficiencies: Poor dietary choices can lead to nutrient deficiencies, causing a range of health problems. For example, a lack of calcium and vitamin D may contribute to bone disorders.

2. Exacerbation of Health Conditions: In conditions like colitis, consuming trigger foods can exacerbate symptoms, leading to increased inflammation and discomfort. Similarly, improper nutrition can accelerate the progression of chronic diseases.

3. Weakened Immune System: Inadequate nutrition compromises the immune system's function, making the body more susceptible to infections and illnesses.

4. Energy Slump: Diets high in processed foods, sugars, and saturated fats can lead to energy slumps, affecting productivity and overall well-being.

5. Increased Risk of Chronic Diseases: Poor dietary habits contribute to the development of chronic diseases such as diabetes, cardiovascular diseases, and obesity.

6. Cognitive Decline: In the context of Alzheimer's and other neurodegenerative diseases, an unhealthy diet may accelerate cognitive decline and impair brain function.

Chapter 1: Delicious Breakfast Recipes

Below are 10 delicious, nutrient-rich, and easy-to-prepare breakfast recipes tailored for the Mediterranean Dash Diet:

1. Mediterranean Veggie Omelette

Ingredients

1. 2 large eggs
2. 1/4 cup cherry tomatoes, halved
3. 1/4 cup spinach, chopped
4. 2 tablespoons feta cheese, crumbled
5. 1 tablespoon olive oil
6. Salt and pepper to taste

Instructions

1. Whisk eggs in a bowl and season with salt and pepper.
2. Heat olive oil in a pan over medium heat.
3. Pour eggs into the pan and add tomatoes, spinach, and feta.
4. Cook until the eggs are set, then fold in half.

5. Serve hot.

Servings: 1

Nutritional Value (per serving)

- Calories: 300
- Protein: 18g
- Healthy fats

2. Greek Yogurt Parfait

Ingredients

1. 1/2 cup Greek yogurt (low-fat)
2. 1/4 cup granola (unsweetened)
3. 1/2 cup mixed berries (blueberries, raspberries)
4. 1 tablespoon honey

Instructions

1. Layer Greek yogurt, granola, and berries in a glass.
2. Drizzle with honey.
3. Repeat for additional layers.
4. Serve chilled.

Servings: 1

Nutritional Value (per serving)

- Calories: 250
- Protein: 15g
- Fiber

3. Mediterranean Avocado Toast

Ingredients

1. 1 slice whole-grain bread
2. 1/2 avocado, mashed
3. 1 tablespoon feta cheese, crumbled
4. 1 teaspoon olive oil
5. Cherry tomatoes, sliced (for garnish)
6. Fresh basil leaves (for garnish)

Instructions

1. Toast the bread slice.
2. Spread mashed avocado on the toast.
3. Sprinkle feta cheese, drizzle olive oil, and garnish with tomatoes and basil.

Servings: 1

Nutritional Value (per serving)

- Calories: 280
- Healthy fats
- Fiber

4. Mediterranean Egg and Spinach Wrap

Ingredients

1. 1 whole-grain wrap
2. 2 large eggs, scrambled
3. 1/2 cup spinach, sautéed

4. 1/4 cup feta cheese, crumbled

5. 1 tablespoon tzatziki sauce

Instructions

1. Cook scrambled eggs and sautéed spinach.

2. Place eggs and spinach on the wrap.

3. Add feta cheese and drizzle with tzatziki sauce.

4. Wrap and serve.

Servings: 1

Nutritional Value (per serving)

- Calories: 320

- Protein: 20g

- Healthy fats

5. Mediterranean Chia Seed Pudding

Ingredients

1. 3 tablespoons chia seeds
2. 1/2 cup almond milk (unsweetened)
3. 1/2 teaspoon vanilla extract
4. 1/4 cup pistachios, chopped
5. 1/4 cup pomegranate seeds

Instructions

1. Combine chia seeds, almond milk, and vanilla extract in a jar. Leave in fridge overnight.
2. In the morning, layer chia pudding with pistachios and pomegranate seeds.
3. Serve chilled.

Servings: 1

Nutritional Value (per serving)

- Calories: 280
- Protein: 8g
- Omega-3 fatty acids

6. Mediterranean Shakshuka

Ingredients

1. 1 tablespoon olive oil
2. 1/2 onion, diced

3. 1 clove garlic, minced
4. 1 bell pepper, diced
5. 1 can (14 oz) crushed tomatoes
6. 2 large eggs
7. 1 teaspoon ground cumin
8. 1 teaspoon paprika
9. Salt and pepper to taste
10. Fresh parsley (for garnish)

Instructions

1. Heat olive oil in a pan and sauté onion, garlic, and bell pepper.
2. Add crushed tomatoes, cumin, paprika, salt, and pepper. Simmer for 10 minutes.
3. Make wells in the sauce and crack eggs into them.
4. Cover and cook until the eggs are set.
5. Garnish with fresh parsley.

Servings: 2

Nutritional Value (per serving)

- Calories: 320
- Protein: 14g
- Healthy fats

7. Mediterranean Quinoa Breakfast Bowl

Ingredients

1. 1/2 cup cooked quinoa
2. 1/4 cup cucumber, diced
3. 1/4 cup cherry tomatoes, halved
4. 2 tablespoons Kalamata olives, sliced
5. 1 tablespoon red onion, finely chopped
6. 1 tablespoon feta cheese, crumbled
7. 1 tablespoon olive oil
8. Fresh oregano (for garnish)

Instructions

1. Mix cooked quinoa, cucumber, tomatoes, olives, red onion, and feta in a bowl.
2. Drizzle with olive oil and garnish with fresh oregano.

Servings: 1

Nutritional Value (per serving)

- Calories: 280
- Protein: 8g
- Fiber

8. Mediterranean Spinach and Feta Muffins

Ingredients

1. 2 cups spinach, chopped
2. 1/2 cup feta cheese, crumbled
3. 1/4 cup sun-dried tomatoes, chopped
4. 4 eggs
5. 1/4 cup whole-wheat flour
6. 1/2 teaspoon baking powder
7. Salt and pepper to taste

Instructions

1. Preheat the oven to 350°F (175°C).
2. In a bowl, mix spinach, feta, and sun-dried tomatoes.
3. In another bowl, whisk eggs, flour, baking powder, salt, and pepper.
4. Combine both mixtures and pour into muffin cups.
5. Bake until set.

Servings: 6

Nutritional Value (per serving)

- Calories: 180
- Protein: 10g
- Healthy fats

9. Mediterranean Fruit Salad

Ingredients

1. 1 cup mixed fruits (grapes, oranges, kiwi)
2. 1/4 cup almonds, sliced
3. 2 tablespoons Greek yogurt (low-fat)
4. 1 tablespoon honey
5. Fresh mint leaves (for garnish)

Instructions

1. Combine mixed fruits in a bowl.
2. Top with sliced almonds, Greek yogurt, and drizzle with honey.
3. Garnish with fresh mint leaves.

Servings: 1

Nutritional Value (per serving)

- Calories: 220
- Protein: 5g
- Fiber

10. Mediterranean Whole Grain Pancakes

Ingredients

1. 1/2 cup whole wheat flour
2. 1/4 cup oats
3. 1/2 teaspoon baking powder

4. 1/2 cup almond milk (unsweetened)

5. 1 egg

6. 1 tablespoon olive oil

7. 1/2 teaspoon vanilla extract

8. Fresh berries (for topping)

Instructions

1. In a bowl, mix whole wheat flour, oats, and baking powder.

2. In another bowl, whisk almond milk, egg, olive oil, and vanilla extract.

3. Combine wet and dry ingredients to form a batter.

4. Cook pancakes on a griddle until golden.

5. Top with fresh berries.

Servings: 2

Nutritional Value (per serving)

- Calories: 220
- Protein: 7g
- Fiber

Chapter 2: Nutrients-Rich Lunch Recipes

Below are 10 delicious, nutrient-rich, and easy-to-prepare lunch recipes tailored for the Mediterranean Dash Diet:

1. Mediterranean Chickpea Salad

Ingredients

1. 1 can (15 oz) chickpeas, drained
2. 1 cucumber, diced
3. 1 cup cherry tomatoes, halved
4. 1/4 cup red onion, finely chopped
5. 1/4 cup Kalamata olives, sliced
6. 2 tablespoons feta cheese, crumbled
7. 2 tablespoons olive oil
8. 1 tablespoon red wine vinegar
9. Fresh oregano (for garnish)

Instructions

1. In a bowl, combine chickpeas, cucumber, tomatoes, red onion, olives, and feta.
2. Mizzle with olive oil and red wine vinegar. Toss gently.
3. Garnish with fresh oregano.
Servings: 2
Nutritional Value (per serving)
- Calories: 300
- Protein: 10g
- Healthy fats

2. Grilled Mediterranean Chicken Wrap

Ingredients
1. 4 oz chicken breast, grilled and sliced
2. 1 whole-grain wrap
3. 1/4 cup hummus
4. 1/4 cup cucumber, julienned
5. 1/4 cup cherry tomatoes, sliced
6. 2 tablespoons feta cheese, crumbled
7. 1 tablespoon tzatziki sauce

Instructions
1. Spread hummus on the wrap.

2. Add grilled chicken, cucumber, tomatoes, feta, and drizzle with tzatziki.

3. Wrap and serve.

Servings: 1

Nutritional Value (per serving)

- Calories: 320
- Protein: 25g
- Healthy fats

3. Mediterranean Quinoa Salad Bowl

Ingredients

1. 1/2 cup cooked quinoa
2. 1/2 cup chickpeas, cooked
3. 1/4 cup red bell pepper, diced
4. 1/4 cup cucumber, diced
5. 2 tablespoons feta cheese, crumbled
6. 1 tablespoon Kalamata olives, sliced
7. 1 tablespoon olive oil
8. 1 tablespoon lemon juice
9. Fresh parsley (for garnish)

Instructions

1. In a bowl, combine quinoa, chickpeas, bell pepper, cucumber, feta, and olives.

2. Drizzle with olive oil and lemon juice.
Toss gently.
3. Garnish with fresh parsley.
Servings: 1
Nutritional Value (per serving)
- Calories: 320
- Protein: 12g
- Healthy fats

4. Mediterranean Lentil Soup

Ingredients
1. 1 cup lentils, rinsed
2. 1 onion, diced
3. 2 carrots, diced
4. 2 celery stalks, diced
5. 3 cloves garlic, minced
6. 1 can (14 oz) diced tomatoes
7. 1 teaspoon cumin
8. 1 teaspoon paprika
9. 4 cups vegetable broth
10. Fresh parsley (for garnish)
Instructions
1. In a pot, sauté onion, carrots, celery, and garlic until softened.

2. Add lentils, tomatoes, cumin, paprika, and vegetable broth.

3. Simmer until lentils are tender.

4. Garnish with fresh parsley.

Servings: 4

Nutritional Value (per serving)

- Calories: 280

- Protein: 18g

- Fiber

5. Mediterranean Stuffed Bell Peppers

Ingredients

1. 2 bell peppers, halved

2. 1 cup cooked quinoa

3. 1/2 cup chickpeas, cooked

4. 1/4 cup red onion, finely chopped

5. 1/4 cup feta cheese, crumbled

6. 1/4 cup cherry tomatoes, diced

7. 2 tablespoons Kalamata olives, sliced

8. 1 tablespoon olive oil

9. 1 teaspoon dried oregano

Instructions

1. Preheat the oven to 375°F (190°C).

2. In a bowl, mix quinoa, chickpeas, red onion, feta, tomatoes, olives, olive oil, and oregano.

3. Stuffed bell pepper halves with the mixture.

4. Bake for 20-25 minutes or until peppers are tender.

Servings: 2

Nutritional Value (per serving)

- Calories: 290
- Protein: 12g
- Healthy fats

6. Mediterranean Shrimp Salad

Ingredients

1. 6 oz shrimp, grilled or sautéed
2. 2 cups mixed greens
3. 1/4 cup cherry tomatoes, halved
4. 1/4 cup cucumber, sliced
5. 1/4 cup red bell pepper, sliced
6. 2 tablespoons feta cheese, crumbled
7. 1 tablespoon olive oil
8. 1 tablespoon balsamic vinegar

Instructions

1. Arrange mixed greens on a plate.

2. Top with grilled shrimp, tomatoes, cucumber, bell pepper, and feta.

3. Spray with olive oil and balsamic vinegar.

Servings: 1

Nutritional Value (per serving)

- Calories: 280
- Protein: 20g
- Healthy fats

7. Mediterranean Eggplant and Chickpea Bowl

Ingredients

1. 1 cup eggplant, diced
2. 1/2 cup chickpeas, cooked
3. 1/4 cup red onion, diced
4. 1/4 cup cherry tomatoes, halved
5. 2 tablespoons feta cheese, crumbled
6. 1 tablespoon olive oil
7. 1 teaspoon dried oregano

Instructions

1. Sauté eggplant, chickpeas, red onion, and cherry tomatoes in olive oil until tender.

2. Sprinkle with feta and oregano.

3. Serve warm.

Servings: 1

Nutritional Value (per serving)

- Calories: 270
- Protein: 9g
- Healthy fats

8. Mediterranean Turkey and Spinach Wrap

Ingredients

1. 4 oz ground turkey, cooked
2. 1 whole-grain wrap
3. 1/4 cup hummus
4. 1/4 cup spinach leaves
5. 1/4 cup cucumber, julienned
6. 1/4 cup tomatoes, diced
7. 1 tablespoon feta cheese, crumbled

Instructions

1. Spread hummus on the wrap.
2. Add cooked ground turkey, spinach, cucumber, tomatoes, and feta.
3. Wrap and serve.

Servings: 1

Nutritional Value (per serving)

- Calories: 320

- Protein: 24g
- Healthy fats

9. Mediterranean Tuna Salad Bowl

Ingredients

1. 1 can (5 oz) tuna, drained
2. 2 cups mixed greens
3. 1/4 cup cucumber, sliced
4. 1/4 cup cherry tomatoes, halved
5. 1/4 cup red onion, thinly sliced
6. 2 tablespoons Kalamata olives, sliced
7. 1 tablespoon olive oil
8. 1 tablespoon lemon juice

Instructions

1. In a bowl, combine tuna, mixed greens, cucumber, tomatoes, red onion, and olives.
2. Drizzle with olive oil and lemon juice. Toss gently.

Servings: 1

Nutritional Value (per serving)

- Calories: 290
- Protein: 25g
- Healthy fats

10. Mediterranean Farro Bowl

Ingredients

1. 1/2 cup cooked farro
2. 1/4 cup chickpeas, cooked
3. 1/4 cup artichoke hearts, chopped
4. 1/4 cup cucumber, diced
5. 2 tablespoons feta cheese, crumbled
6. 1 tablespoon olive oil
7. 1 tablespoon balsamic vinegar
8. Fresh mint leaves (for garnish)

Instructions

1. Combine cooked farro, chickpeas, artichoke hearts, cucumber, and feta in a bowl.
2. Drizzle with olive oil and balsamic vinegar. Toss gently.
3. Garnish with fresh mint leaves.

Servings: 1

Nutritional Value (per serving)

- Calories: 310
- Protein: 12g
- Healthy fats

Chapter 3: Satisfying Dinner Recipes

Below are 10 delicious, nutrient-rich, and easy-to-prepare dinner recipes tailored for the Mediterranean Dash Diet:

1. Mediterranean Baked Salmon

Ingredients

1. 2 salmon filets (6 oz each)
2. 1 tablespoon olive oil
3. 1 lemon, sliced
4. 2 cloves garlic, minced
5. 1 teaspoon dried oregano
6. 1 teaspoon paprika
7. Salt and pepper to taste

Instructions

1. Preheat the oven to 400°F (200°C).
2. Place salmon filets on a baking sheet.
3. Drizzle with olive oil, sprinkle garlic, oregano, paprika, salt, and pepper.
4. Top with lemon slices.
5. Bake until the salmon is cooked.

Servings: 2

Nutritional Value (per serving)
- Calories: 320
- Protein: 30g
- Omega-3 fatty acids

2. Mediterranean Quinoa Stuffed Peppers

Ingredients
1. 4 bell peppers, halved
2. 1 cup cooked quinoa
3. 1/2 cup cherry tomatoes, diced
4. 1/4 cup Kalamata olives, sliced
5. 1/4 cup feta cheese, crumbled
6. 2 tablespoons fresh parsley, chopped
7. 1 tablespoon olive oil
8. 1 teaspoon dried oregano

Instructions
1. Preheat the oven to 375°F (190°C).
2. In a bowl, mix quinoa, tomatoes, olives, feta, parsley, olive oil, and oregano.
3. Stuffed bell pepper halves with the mixture.
4. Bake for 25-30 minutes.

Servings: 4

Nutritional Value (per serving)
- Calories: 260
- Protein: 10g
- Fiber

3. Mediterranean Vegetable Skewers

Ingredients
1. 1 zucchini, sliced
2. 1 eggplant, diced
3. 1 red bell pepper, diced
4. 1 yellow bell pepper, diced
5. 1 red onion, sliced
6. 8 cherry tomatoes
7. 1/4 cup olive oil
8. 2 tablespoons balsamic vinegar
9. 1 teaspoon dried basil
10. Salt and pepper to taste

Instructions
1. Preheat the grill.
2. Thread vegetables onto skewers.
3. In a bowl, whisk olive oil, balsamic vinegar, basil, salt, and pepper.
4. Grill skewers for 10-15 minutes, turning occasionally.

Servings: 4

Nutritional Value (per serving)
- Calories: 180
- Healthy fats
- Fiber

4. Mediterranean Chickpea and Spinach Stew

Ingredients

1. 1 can (15 oz) chickpeas, drained
2. 1 onion, diced
3. 2 cloves garlic, minced
4. 1 can (14 oz) diced tomatoes
5. 4 cups spinach
6. 1 teaspoon cumin
7. 1 teaspoon paprika
8. 1/4 cup feta cheese, crumbled
9. 2 tablespoons olive oil

Instructions

1. In a pot, sauté onion and garlic in olive oil until softened.
2. Add chickpeas, tomatoes, cumin, paprika, and simmer for 15 minutes.
3. Stir in spinach until wilted.
4. Top with feta before serving.

Servings: 4

Nutritional Value (per serving)
- Calories: 250
- Protein: 10g
- Healthy fats

5. Mediterranean Turkey Meatballs

Ingredients
1. 1 lb ground turkey
2. 1/2 cup whole-wheat breadcrumbs
3. 1/4 cup fresh parsley, chopped
4. 1/4 cup feta cheese, crumbled
5. 1 egg
6. 2 cloves garlic, minced
7. 1 teaspoon dried oregano
8. Salt and pepper to taste
9. 1 can (14 oz) diced tomatoes

Instructions
1. Preheat the oven to 375°F (190°C).
2. In a bowl, mix turkey, breadcrumbs, parsley, feta, egg, garlic, oregano, salt, and pepper.
3. Form into meatballs and place on a baking sheet.
4. Bake for 20-25 minutes.
5. Serve over diced tomatoes.

Servings: 4
Nutritional Value (per serving)
- Calories: 280
- Protein: 25g
- Healthy fats

6. Mediterranean Shrimp and Quinoa Bowl

Ingredients

1. 1 cup cooked quinoa
2. 6 oz shrimp, grilled or sautéed
3. 1/2 cup cherry tomatoes, halved
4. 1/4 cup Kalamata olives, sliced
5. 2 tablespoons feta cheese, crumbled
6. 1 tablespoon olive oil
7. 1 tablespoon lemon juice
8. Fresh basil leaves (for garnish)

Instructions

1. In a bowl, combine quinoa, shrimp, tomatoes, olives, and feta.
2. Drizzle with olive oil and lemon juice. Toss gently.
3. Garnish with fresh basil.

Servings: 2
Nutritional Value (per serving)

- Calories: 320
- Protein: 20g
- Healthy fats

7. Mediterranean Stuffed Zucchini Boats

Ingredients

1. 2 large zucchini, halved
2. 1 cup cooked farro
3. 1/2 cup cherry tomatoes, diced
4. 1/4 cup feta cheese, crumbled
5. 1/4 cup Kalamata olives, sliced
6. 1 tablespoon olive oil
7. 1 teaspoon dried oregano

Instructions

1. Preheat the oven to 375°F (190°C).
2. Scoop out the center of each zucchini half.
3. In a bowl, mix farro, tomatoes, feta, olives, olive oil, and oregano.
4. Stuff zucchini with the mixture.
5. Bake for 20-25 minutes.

Servings: 4

Nutritional Value (per serving)

- Calories: 260

- Protein: 8g
- Healthy fats

8. Mediterranean Chicken and Vegetable Skillet

Ingredients

1. 2 chicken breasts, sliced
2. 1 cup cherry tomatoes, halved
3. 1 zucchini, sliced
4. 1 yellow bell pepper, sliced
5. 1/4 cup black olives, sliced
6. 2 tablespoons olive oil
7. 1 teaspoon dried basil
8. Salt and pepper to taste

Instructions

1. Season chicken with salt and pepper.
2. In a skillet, heat olive oil and cook chicken until browned.
3. Add tomatoes, zucchini, bell pepper, and olives. Sauté until vegetables are tender.
4. Sprinkle with dried basil before serving.

Servings: 2

Nutritional Value (per serving)
- Calories: 330
- Protein: 30g
- Healthy fats

9. Mediterranean Eggplant and Lentil Casserole

Ingredients
1. 1 large eggplant, sliced
2. 1 cup cooked lentils
3. 1 can (14 oz) diced tomatoes
4. 1/4 cup feta cheese, crumbled
5. 2 cloves garlic, minced
6. 1 teaspoon dried oregano
7. 2 tablespoons olive oil

Instructions
1. Preheat the oven to 375°F (190°C).
2. In a casserole dish, layer eggplant, lentils, tomatoes, feta, garlic, and oregano.
3. Repeat the layers.
4. Drizzle with olive oil.
5. Bake for at least 30-35 minutes.

Servings: 4

Nutritional Value (per serving)

- Calories: 280
- Protein: 14g
- Healthy fats

10. Mediterranean Cauliflower Rice Bowl

Ingredients

1. 2 cups cauliflower rice, cooked
2. 1/2 cup chickpeas, cooked
3. 1/4 cup cucumber, diced
4. 1/4 cup cherry tomatoes, halved
5. 2 tablespoons Kalamata olives, sliced
6. 1 tablespoon feta cheese, crumbled
7. 1 tablespoon olive oil
8. 1 tablespoon lemon juice
9. Fresh mint leaves (for garnish)

Instructions

1. In a bowl, combine cauliflower rice, chickpeas, cucumber, tomatoes, olives, and feta.
2. Drizzle with olive oil and lemon juice. Toss gently.
3. Garnish with fresh mint.

Servings: 2

Nutritional Value (per serving)

- Calories: 240
- Protein: 10g
- Healthy fats

Chapter 4: Easy-to-prepare Snacks and Dessert Recipes

Below are 10 delicious, nutrient-rich, and easy-to-prepare snacks and dessert recipes tailored for the Mediterranean Dash Diet:

1. Mediterranean Hummus Platter

Ingredients

1. 1 cup hummus
2. 1/4 cup cherry tomatoes, halved
3. 1/4 cup cucumber, sliced
4. 1/4 cup Kalamata olives, sliced
5. 1 tablespoon olive oil
6. Whole-grain pita bread (for serving)

Instructions

1. Spread hummus on a serving platter.
2. Arrange tomatoes, cucumber, and olives on top.
3. Drizzle with olive oil.
4. Serve with whole-grain pita bread.

Servings: 4

Nutritional Value (per serving)
- Calories: 180
- Protein: 5g
- Healthy fats

2. Mediterranean Yogurt Parfait

Ingredients
1. 1 cup Greek yogurt (low-fat)
2. 1/4 cup granola
3. 1/4 cup mixed berries (blueberries, strawberries)
4. 1 tablespoon honey
5. Chopped mint leaves (for garnish)

Instructions
1. In a glass cup, lay out Greek yogurt, granola, and mixed berries.
2. Drizzle with honey.
3. Garnish with chopped mint.

Servings: 2

Nutritional Value (per serving)
- Calories: 200
- Protein: 15g
- Fiber

3. Mediterranean Fruit Kabobs

Ingredients

1. 1 cup watermelon, cubed
2. 1 cup cantaloupe, cubed
3. 1 cup pineapple, cubed
4. 1/4 cup mint leaves, chopped
5. Wooden skewers

Instructions

1. Thread watermelon, cantaloupe, and pineapple on wooden skewers.
2. Sprinkle with chopped mint.
3. Chill before serving.

Servings: 4

Nutritional Value (per serving)

- Calories: 60
- Vitamin C

4. Mediterranean Dark Chocolate-Dipped Strawberries

Ingredients

1. 1 cup strawberries, washed and dried
2. 1/4 cup dark chocolate, melted
3. Chopped pistachios (optional)

Instructions

1. Dip each strawberry in melted dark chocolate.

2. Place on parchment paper.

3. Sprinkle with chopped pistachios if desired.

4. Allow chocolate to set.

Servings: 4

Nutritional Value (per serving)

- Calories: 50

- Antioxidants

5. Mediterranean Energy Bites

Ingredients

1. 1 cup almonds

2. 1 cup dates, pitted

3. 1 tablespoon chia seeds

4. 1 teaspoon cinnamon

5. 1/4 cup shredded coconut (unsweetened)

Instructions

1. In a food processor, blend almonds, dates, chia seeds, and cinnamon until a sticky dough forms.

2. Roll into bite-sized balls and coat with shredded coconut.

3. Chill before serving.

Servings: 8

Nutritional Value (per serving)

- Calories: 120
- Protein: 3g
- Healthy fats

6. Mediterranean Greek Yogurt Bark

Ingredients

1. 2 cups Greek yogurt (low-fat)
2. 1/4 cup honey
3. 1/4 cup mixed berries (blueberries, raspberries)
4. 2 tablespoons pistachios, chopped

Instructions

1. In a bowl, mingle Greek yogurt and honey.
2. Spread the mixture on a parchment-lined tray.
3. Sprinkle with mixed berries and chopped pistachios.
4. Freeze until firm, then break into pieces.

Servings: 4

Nutritional Value (per serving)

- Calories: 150
- Protein: 10g
- Healthy fats

7. Mediterranean Roasted Chickpeas

Ingredients

1. 1 can (15 oz) chickpeas, drained and rinsed
2. 1 tablespoon olive oil
3. 1 teaspoon cumin
4. 1/2 teaspoon smoked paprika
5. Sea salt to taste

Instructions

1. Preheat the oven to 400°F (200°C).
2. Pat chickpeas dry and toss with olive oil, cumin, paprika, and salt.
3. Roast for 25-30 minutes, stirring halfway.

Servings: 4

Nutritional Value (per serving)

- Calories: 120
- Protein: 5g
- Fiber

8. Mediterranean Apple Nachos

Ingredients

1. 1 apple, thinly sliced
2. 2 tablespoons almond butter (unsweetened)
3. 1 tablespoon honey
4. 1 tablespoon pomegranate seeds
5. 1 tablespoon chopped walnuts

Instructions

1. Arrange apple slices on a plate.
2. Drizzle with almond butter and honey.
3. Sprinkle with pomegranate seeds and chopped walnuts.

Servings: 2

Nutritional Value (per serving)

- Calories: 150
- Fiber
- Healthy fats

9. Mediterranean Berry Sorbet

Ingredients

1. 2 cups of different berries (strawberries, blueberries, raspberries)
2. 1 tablespoon honey
3. 1 tablespoon lemon juice
4. Fresh mint leaves (for garnish)

Instructions

1. In a blender, puree mixed berries, honey, and lemon juice.
2. Pour into a shallow dish and freeze for 4 hours, stirring occasionally.
3. Scoop into bowls and garnish with fresh mint.

Servings: 4

Nutritional Value (per serving)

- Calories: 50
- Vitamin C

10. Mediterranean Pistachio Biscotti

Ingredients

1. 1 cup whole-wheat flour
2. 1/2 cup almond flour
3. 1/4 cup honey
4. Zest of 1 orange

5. 1/4 cup pistachios, chopped
6. 1 egg
7. 1/2 teaspoon baking powder
Instructions
1. Preheat the oven to 350°F (175°C).
2. In a bowl, mix whole-wheat flour, almond flour, honey, orange zest, pistachios, egg, and baking powder.
3. Shape the dough into a log and bake for 20-25 minutes.
4. Allow to cool, then slice into biscotti.
Servings: 8
Nutritional Value (per serving)
- Calories: 120
- Protein: 3g
- Healthy fats

Chapter 5: Bonus 1

20 Juicing and Smoothie Recipes

1. Mediterranean Citrus Bliss Juice

Ingredients

1. 2 oranges, peeled
2. 1 grapefruit, peeled
3. 1 lemon, peeled

Instructions

1. Juice the oranges, grapefruit, and lemon.
2. Stir well and serve over ice.

2. Green Goddess Detox Juice

Ingredients

1. 1 cucumber
2. 2 celery stalks
3. 1 cup spinach
4. 1/2 lemon, peeled

Instructions

1. Juice the cucumber, celery, spinach, and lemon.
2. Mix well and enjoy.

3. Antioxidant Berry Blast

Ingredients

1. 1 cup mixed berries (blueberries, raspberries, strawberries)
2. 1/2 cup pomegranate seeds
3. 1/2 cup water

Instructions

1. Blend the mixed berries, pomegranate seeds, and water until smooth.
2. Pour into a glass and enjoy.

4. Turmeric Tonic

Ingredients

1. 1 apple, cored and sliced
2. 1/2 inch ginger, peeled
3. 1/2 teaspoon turmeric powder
4. 1 cup coconut water

Instructions

1. Juice the apple and ginger.
2. Stir in turmeric powder and coconut water.
3. Mix well and serve.

5. Cucumber Mint Cooler

Ingredients

1. 2 cucumbers
2. 1/4 cup fresh mint leaves
3. 1/2 lime, peeled

Instructions

1. Juice the cucumbers, mint leaves, and lime.
2. Chill and serve over ice.

6. Pineapple Basil Delight

Ingredients

1. 1 cup pineapple chunks
2. 1/4 cup fresh basil leaves
3. 1/2 lemon, peeled

Instructions

1. Blend the pineapple chunks, basil leaves, and lemon until smooth.
2. Pour into a glass and enjoy.

7. Carrot Orange Sunshine

Ingredients

1. 4 carrots, peeled
2. 2 oranges, peeled
3. 1/2 inch turmeric, peeled

Instructions

1. Juice the carrots, oranges, and turmeric.
2. Mix well and serve over ice.

8. Beetroot Berry Blast

Ingredients

1. 1 medium-sized beetroot, peeled
2. 1 cup mixed berries (blueberries, raspberries, strawberries)
3. 1/2 cup water

Instructions

1. Juice the beetroot and mixed berries.
2. Dilute with water, stir, and enjoy.

9. Mediterranean Green Goddess Smoothie

Ingredients

1. 1 cup kale

2. 1/2 cucumber

3. 1/2 avocado

4. 1/2 lemon, peeled

5. 1 cup coconut water

Instructions

1. Blend the kale, cucumber, avocado, lemon, and coconut water until smooth.

2. Pour into a glass and enjoy.

10. Berry Bliss Smoothie

Ingredients

1. 1 cup mixed berries (blueberries, raspberries, strawberries)

2. 1/2 cup Greek yogurt (low-fat)

3. 1 tablespoon chia seeds

4. 1/2 cup almond milk

Instructions

1. Blend the mixed berries, Greek yogurt, chia seeds, and almond milk until smooth.

2. Pour into a glass and savor.

11. Mango Tango Smoothie

Ingredients

1. 1 cup mango chunks
2. 1/2 banana
3. 1/2 cup spinach
4. 1/2 cup water

Instructions

1. Blend the mango chunks, banana, spinach, and water until smooth.
2. Pour into a glass and enjoy.

12. Pomegranate Paradise Smoothie

Ingredients

1. 1/2 cup pomegranate seeds
2. 1/2 cup pineapple chunks
3. 1/2 cup Greek yogurt (low-fat)
4. 1/2 cup water

Instructions

1. Blend the pomegranate seeds, pineapple chunks, Greek yogurt, and water until smooth.
2. Pour into a glass and savor.

13. Minty Pineapple Refresher

Ingredients

1. 1 cup pineapple chunks
2. 1/4 cup fresh mint leaves

3. 1/2 lime, peeled

4. 1/2 cucumber

Instructions

1. Juice the pineapple chunks, mint leaves, lime, and cucumber.

2. Mix well and serve over ice.

14. Green Apple Ginger Zinger

Ingredients

1. 2 green apples, cored and sliced

2. 1/2 inch ginger, peeled

3. 1 cup spinach

4. 1/2 cup coconut water

Instructions

1. Blend the green apples, ginger, spinach, and coconut water until smooth.

2. Pour into a glass and savor.

15. Citrus Avocado Dream Smoothie

Ingredients

1. 1 orange, peeled

2. 1/2 grapefruit, peeled

3. 1/2 avocado

4. 1 tablespoon chia seeds
5. 1/2 cup water
Instructions
1. Blend the orange, grapefruit, avocado, chia seeds, and water until smooth.
2. Pour into a glass and enjoy.

16. Blueberry Almond Bliss Smoothie

Ingredients
1. 1 cup blueberries
2. 1/2 cup almonds, soaked
3. 1/2 cup Greek yogurt (low-fat)
4. 1/2 cup almond milk
Instructions:
1. Blend the blueberries, soaked almonds, Greek yogurt, and almond milk until smooth.
2. Pour into a glass and savor.

17. Cucumber Melon Refresher

Ingredients
1. 1 cup cucumber, sliced
2. 1 cup honeydew melon, cubed

3. 1/4 cup fresh mint leaves

4. 1/2 lime, peeled

Instructions

1. Blend the cucumber, honeydew melon, mint leaves, and lime until smooth.

2. Pour into a glass and enjoy.

18. Carrot Mango Tango

Ingredients

1. 2 carrots, peeled and sliced

2. 1 cup mango chunks

3. 1/2 banana

4. 1/2 cup water

Instructions

1. Blend the carrots, mango chunks, banana, and water until smooth.

2. Pour into a glass and savor.

19. Peachy Green Smoothie

Ingredients

1. 1 cup peaches, sliced

2. 1 cup kale

3. 1/2 cup Greek yogurt (low-fat)

4. 1/2 cup water

Instructions

1. Blend the peaches, kale, Greek yogurt, and water until smooth.

2. Pour into a glass and enjoy.

20. Cherry Almond Delight Smoothie

Ingredients

1. 1 cup cherries, pitted
2. 1/2 cup almonds, soaked
3. 1/2 cup Greek yogurt (low-fat)
4. 1/2 cup almond milk

Instructions

1. Blend the cherries, soaked almonds, Greek yogurt, and almond milk until smooth.

2. Pour into a glass and savor.

Conclusion

This Mediterranean Dash Diet cookbook for seniors offers a flavorful journey toward improved health and well-being.

With a focus on nutrient-rich ingredients, delicious recipes, and scientifically proven approaches, this collection provides a practical guide for embracing the Mediterranean Dash Diet lifestyle. By incorporating these culinary delights into your daily routine, you're not only savoring vibrant flavors but also nourishing your body with the essential nutrients it craves. Let this cookbook be your companion on the path to a healthier and more enjoyable way of eating, proving that wholesome nutrition can indeed be a delightful journey. Here's to a healthier you through the nourishing embrace of the Mediterranean Dash Diet!